Contents

Introduction

My Struggle with weight and what I've learned.

As a child, I began to get a little chubby around the middle. I didn't have a problem with it. I didn't think there was a problem actually, and I didn't have a care about it. I was just trying to be a happy normal kid.

Being around other kids that teased me for being a bit chubby wasn't easy to deal with. It made me feel really insecure about my appearance. Once I became an adult, I grew to a height of 5 ft 1 in. which is more on the petite side than tall, and gaining just a few extra pounds on my small frame, looked like a lot of weight. Although I was an adult now, I still felt the same insecurity with my weight, and this lack of confidence stuck with me as I got older. Many years later I learned that I was not the only one that struggled with weight, and this is something a lot of teens and adults go through.

There were times when I tried really strict diets, like only allowing myself 500 calories a day, and then feeling so deprived that it always led to binge eating or giving in to cravings for cake and cookies. It was tough because I didn't really know what to eat, or how much.

A lot of the diets out there wouldn't appeal to me because the food menu they would provide didn't have choices I could eat as I have a problem with milk products.

I believed that if I just kept my calories low, I'd lose weight, but it turns out weight loss doesn't work that way.

I would do the 500 calorie diet, along with workouts and I would lose some weight. I would even go to extremes of eating once a day and exercising constantly, which looking back seems crazy! Sure, I'd lose some weight doing that, but it wasn't sustainable. Eventually, I'd go back to indulging in my favorite foods and gain the weight back.

I also tried diet pills back then, because they were everywhere in ads promising quick weight loss. Some of them did seem to work a bit, by curbing your appetite. That was not a healthy approach for me. I feel that a diet pill that provides vitamins and ingredients to help the body turn food into energy would have been a better choice.

There were times I've done well and felt great, but other times I've felt really disappointed. I've learned a lot from trying different approaches with dieting and doing research to find answers.

In this book, I want to talk about things I've figured out along the way that have made a huge difference in how I manage my weight now. These aren't just tips; they're real strategies that have completely changed how I manage my weight and incorporated a healthy lifestyle.

So come along with me as I share the strategies that have helped me transform how I eat, exercise, and feel about myself.

Chapter 1

Being Overweight and Obesity

Why are people overweight?

There isn't a single, straightforward answer to why people become overweight, as it's a complex issue influenced by various factors. Here are some common reasons:

Poor Diet: Consuming high-calorie, low-nutrient foods like processed snacks, sugary drinks, and fast food can contribute to weight gain.

Lack of Physical Activity: Sedentary lifestyles, characterized by long periods of sitting and minimal exercise, can lead to weight gain and obesity.

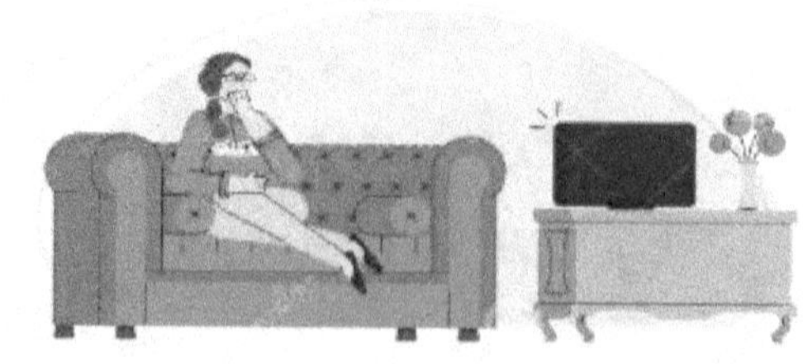

Genetics: Genetics play a role in determining an individual's susceptibility to weight gain and obesity. Some people may have a genetic predisposition that makes it easier for them to gain weight.

Environmental Factors: Environmental factors such as easy access to unhealthy food options, urbanization, and neighborhood safety can influence dietary habits and physical activity levels.

Emotional Factors: Emotional eating, stress, depression, and anxiety can all contribute to overeating and weight gain.

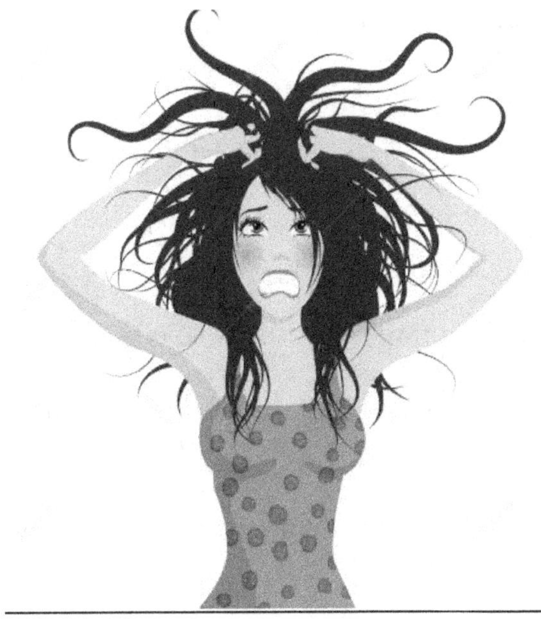

Medical Conditions: Certain medical conditions and medications can lead to weight gain or make it difficult to lose weight, such as hypothyroidism, polycystic ovary syndrome (PCOS), and some antidepressants.

Lack of Sleep: Inadequate sleep or poor sleep quality can disrupt hormonal balance, leading to increased appetite and weight gain.

Social and Cultural Factors: Cultural norms, social pressures, and family habits can all influence eating behaviors and contribute to weight gain.

Marketing and Advertising: Aggressive marketing of unhealthy foods and beverages, coupled with misleading advertising, can influence consumer choices and contribute to overconsumption of calorie-dense foods.

Lifestyle Factors: Busy schedules, long work hours, and lack of time for meal preparation or exercise can make it challenging to maintain a healthy lifestyle.

We can see here that weight gain has many different ways a person can gain weight, and addressing it often requires a holistic approach that considers individual circumstances and challenges.

Activities and Exercise

Why are these so important?

Physical activity and adequate sleep play crucial roles in promoting weight loss through various mechanisms:

Physical activity increases the number of calories your body burns, aiding in creating a calorie deficit necessary for weight loss. Activities such as cardio exercises, strength training, and even daily movement like walking contribute to energy usage. When you engage in physical activity, your muscles require energy, which is obtained from the calories stored in your body. The intensity and duration of the activity determine the number of calories burned.

Cardio exercises, such as running, cycling, or swimming, elevate your heart rate and breathing, resulting in significant calorie usage. These activities not only burn calories during the workout but can also lead to an elevated metabolic rate afterward, known as the after burn effect or excess post-exercise oxygen consumption (EPOC). This means you continue to burn calories at an increased rate even after you've finished exercising.

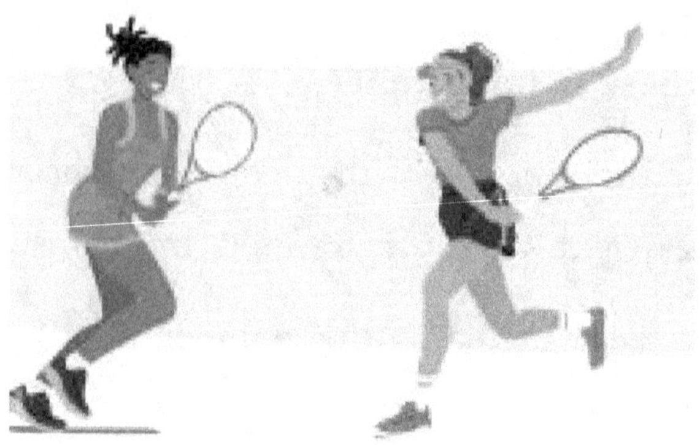

In addition to workouts, daily movement and activities like walking, gardening, or household chores also contribute to energy usage. These low-intensity activities, known as non-exercise activity thermo genesis (NEAT), can add up throughout the day and play a significant role in overall calorie usage.

By incorporating a combination of cardio exercises, strength training, and daily movement into your routine, you can maximize calorie usage; you can accelerate weight loss, and improve overall health and fitness levels.

Metabolism Boost:

Regular physical activity can increase your metabolic rate, meaning your body burns more calories throughout the day, even when you're not exercising. This effect can persist for hours after your workout, depending on the intensity and duration of the activity.

Appetite Regulation:

Exercise can help regulate appetite hormones, such as ghrelin and leptin, which control feelings of hunger and fullness. Some studies suggest that regular exercise may reduce appetite and cravings, making it easier to stick to a calorie-controlled diet. Physical activity enhances insulin sensitivity, allowing your body to more effectively regulates blood sugar levels. This can help prevent spikes in blood sugar and insulin, which are associated with fat storage and weight gain.

Stress and Sleep

Stress Reduction: Exercise is known to reduce stress levels by stimulating the production of endorphins, which are natural mood elevators. Lower stress levels can help prevent emotional eating and reduce the risk of weight gain associated with having a stressful lifestyle which a lot of people have.

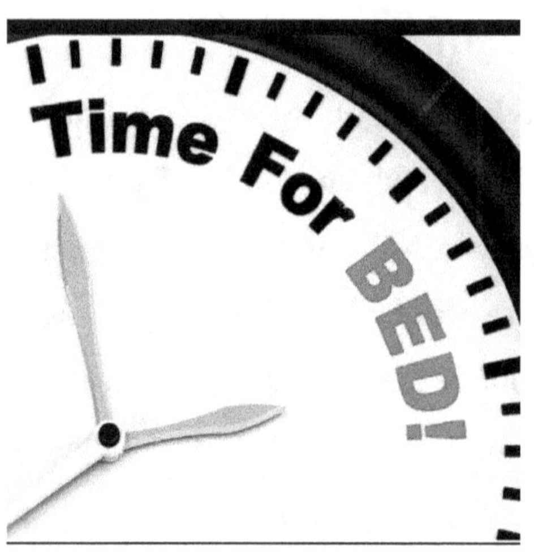

Quality Sleep: Getting enough sleep is essential for overall health, including weight management. Poor sleep can disrupt hormone levels, increasing hunger and appetite while reducing feelings of fullness. It can also lead to higher levels of cortisol, a stress hormone that promotes fat storage, particularly around the abdomen. Not getting enough sleep has been linked to alterations in hormones that regulate hunger and appetite, such as ghrelin and leptin. Lack of sleep can increase ghrelin levels (which stimulate appetite) the reason it stimulates the appetite is because the body needs more food to maintain body strength due to the lack of sleep. This will decrease lepton levels, which suppresses appetite, leading to overeating throughout the day and more weight gain.

I know people who only get about 4 to 5 hours of sleep a night. They say, "I will sleep later," but that doesn't happen because they have developed a habit of not sleeping.

By adding regular physical activity and prioritizing quality sleep into your lifestyle, you can promote your body's ability to burn calories, regulate appetite, and support your weight loss efforts.

Chapter 2

Nutrition

What is Food

Food is Nutritious foods that provide essential nutrients, vitamins, and minerals necessary for optimal bodily function while supporting overall health and well-being. Here are some characteristics of healthy foods.

Healthy Foods come from nature. Healthy foods are rich in nutrients relative to their calorie content. They provide essential vitamins, minerals, fiber, and antioxidants without excessive amounts of added sugars, unhealthy fats, or refined carbohydrates.

A balanced diet includes a variety of foods from different food groups, such as fruits, vegetables, whole grains, lean proteins, and healthy fats. Each food group offers unique nutrients that are essential for various bodily functions.

Fiber is important for digestive health, promoting satiety, and regulating blood sugar levels. Healthy foods like fruits, vegetables, whole grains, legumes, nuts, and seeds are excellent sources of dietary fiber.

Healthy foods contain minimal added sugars. Instead, they derive their sweetness from natural sources like fruits or contain no added sugars at all. Excessive sugar consumption is linked to various health issues, including obesity, type 2 diabetes, and heart disease.

 Healthy foods are low in unhealthy fats, such as saturated and Trans fats, which can increase the risk of heart disease and other health problems. Instead, they contain healthy fats, such as monounsaturated and polyunsaturated fats, found in foods like nuts, seeds, avocados, and fatty fish.

Healthy foods are free of artificial additives, preservatives, colors, and flavors. They contain ingredients that are recognizable and pronounceable, without artificial chemicals or synthetic substances.

Healthy foods can contribute to hydration, as many fruits and vegetables have high water content. Having hydration is essential for overall health and helps support various bodily functions including skin

Examples of healthy foods include:

- Fruits and vegetables

- Whole grains like whole grain bread, brown rice, quinoa, and oats

- Lean proteins such as poultry, fish, tofu, and legumes

- Nuts, seeds, and nut butter

- Healthy fats like olive oil, avocado, and fatty fish (salmon, tuna)

- Dairy or dairy alternatives (unsweetened)

- Herbs, spices, and natural flavorings

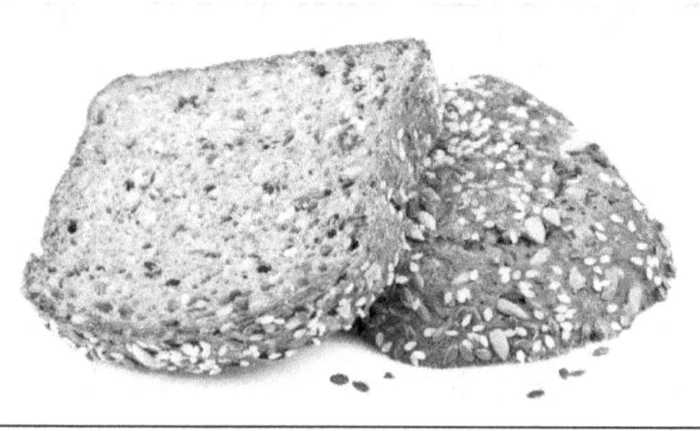

One dietary change I made was eliminating dairy. This was my personal preference. While dairy products are known for their calcium content, they can also be high in fats that contribute to weight gain. Cheese, for example, is dense in both calories and fat. Consider popular dishes like pizza, lasagna, quesadillas, and macaroni and cheese—many of which prominently feature cheese. Just TWO slices of pizza can account for half of your daily calorie intake!   I want to eat more food than just two slices of pizza!

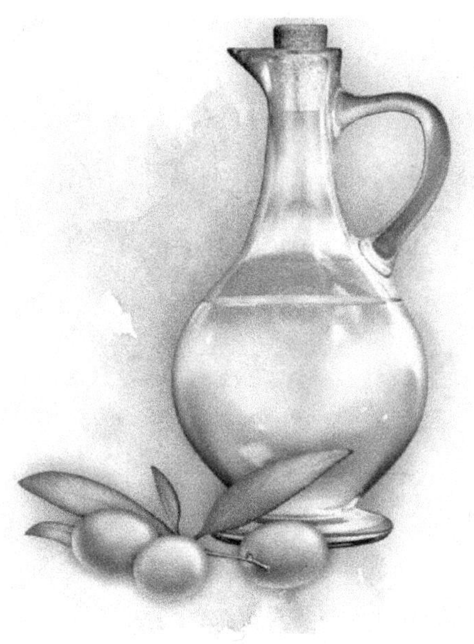

While sour cream undoubtedly enhances the flavor of a potato, its addition can transform an otherwise healthy food choice into a high-fat, high-calorie dish. However, choosing to enjoy the potato without sour cream allows me to fully savor its natural taste without the added fats and calories. Also by doing this, if I'm still hungry, I can have another serving of something else.

Foods to Avoid:

Foods that are often stripped of nutrients and loaded with additives, preservatives, and unhealthy ingredients are foods to avoid.

Avoiding certain foods can help promote overall health and prevent various health issues. Here are some examples of foods that are generally considered unhealthy and best avoided or consumed in moderation like:

INFLAMMATORY FOODS

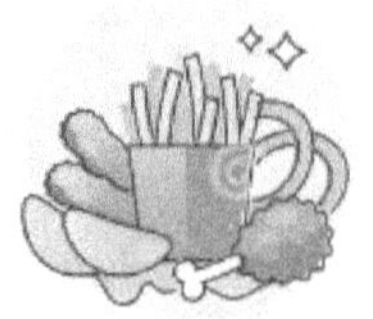

FRIED FOODS

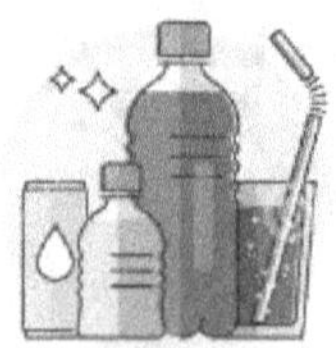

SODAS

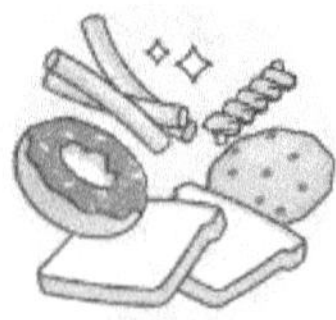

REFINED CARBS

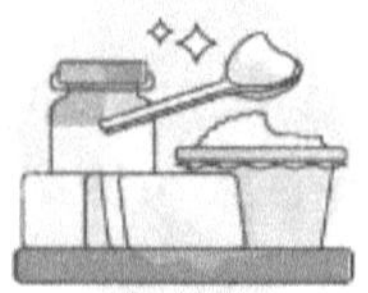

LARD

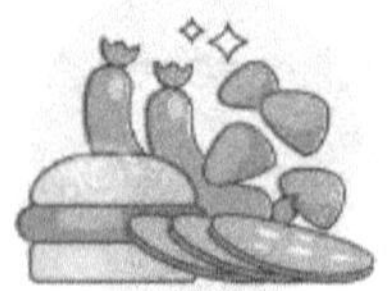

PROCESSED MEATS

Processed Foods: Foods that are processed undergo extensive processing, often containing added sugars, unhealthy fats, preservatives, and artificial additives. Examples include sugary cereals, packaged snacks, frozen meals, and fast food items.

Sugar-Sweetened Beverages: Beverages like soda, fruit drinks, energy drinks, sweetened teas, and flavored coffee drinks are loaded with added sugars and provide little to no nutritional value. They contribute to weight gain, type 2 diabetes, heart disease, and other health problems.

Trans Fats: Trans fats are artificial fats found in partially hydrogenated oils used in processed foods like fried foods, baked goods, margarine, and some packaged snacks. They raise LDL (bad) cholesterol levels and increase the risk of heart disease.

Highly Processed Meats: Processed meats such as bacon, sausage, hot dogs, deli meats, and certain canned meats contain additives, preservatives, and high amounts of sodium. Regular consumption is associated with an increased risk of heart disease, cancer, and other health issues. I have made the choice to not eat these processed meats.

Refined Carbohydrates: Refined carbohydrates are grains that have been stripped of their fiber, vitamins, and minerals during processing. Examples include white bread, white rice, pasta, pastries, and sugary cereals. These foods can cause blood sugar spikes, contribute to weight gain, and increase the risk of type 2 diabetes. I do have some refined carbs on occasion, but not regularly.

Deep-Fried Foods: Foods that are deep-fried in unhealthy oils are high in calories, unhealthy fats, and potentially harmful compounds formed during the frying process. Examples include French fries, fried chicken, doughnuts, and fried snacks. I do have some fried things on occasion, but not regularly.

Highly Sweetened Snacks and Desserts:

Snacks and desserts like candy bars, cookies, cakes, pastries, ice cream, and sweetened yogurt are loaded with added sugars and unhealthy fats. They provide empty calories and can contribute to weight gain and metabolic disorders. Every so often, I will have a cookie or a slice of cake. When I do, the taste is so sweet I can never eat it but half.

Artificial Sweeteners:

While marketed as low-calorie alternatives to sugar, artificial sweeteners like aspartame, sucralose, and saccharin may have negative effects on health and metabolism. It's best to limit consumption and opt for natural sweeteners like stevia or honey instead. I do not use artificial sweeteners at all.

High-Sodium Foods:

Foods high in sodium, such as processed meats, canned soups, salty snacks, and fast food items, can contribute to high blood pressure, heart disease, and stroke. Limiting sodium intake is essential for overall health. When I purchase canned foods I choose Low Sodium. I try to avoid eating canned foods.

Alcohol:

Excessive alcohol consumption poses various health risks, including elevated triglyceride levels due to its high sugar content, potentially leading to heart disease. Moreover, it can adversely affect other organs. Thus, limiting alcohol intake is vital for overall health and well-being. While I recognize moderate alcohol consumption may be acceptable, I have chosen to remove alcohol entirely from my diet.

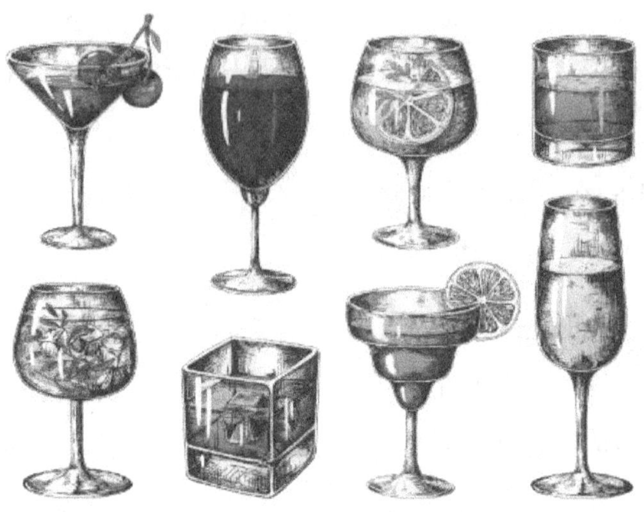

By minimizing or avoiding these unhealthy

Foods, and focusing on whole, nutrient-dense options, you can improve your overall health and reduce the risk of chronic diseases.

Fiber

Fiber like whole grains and whole grain bread is made from grains that include all parts of the kernel. This means it retains valuable nutrients such as fiber, vitamins (like B vitamins), minerals (such as iron and magnesium), and antioxidants. These nutrients are essential for overall health and well-being.

Whole grains and whole grain bread is an excellent source of dietary fiber. Fiber is crucial for digestive health, as it promotes regular bowel movements, prevents constipation, and supports a healthy gut micro biome. Additionally, fiber helps regulate blood sugar levels by slowing down the absorption of glucose, which can reduce the risk of type 2 diabetes.

The fiber in whole grains is particularly beneficial for heart health. It helps lower LDL (bad) cholesterol levels, reduce the risk of cardiovascular disease, and improve overall heart health. Fiber also helps lower blood pressure and triglyceride levels, further supporting cardiovascular health.

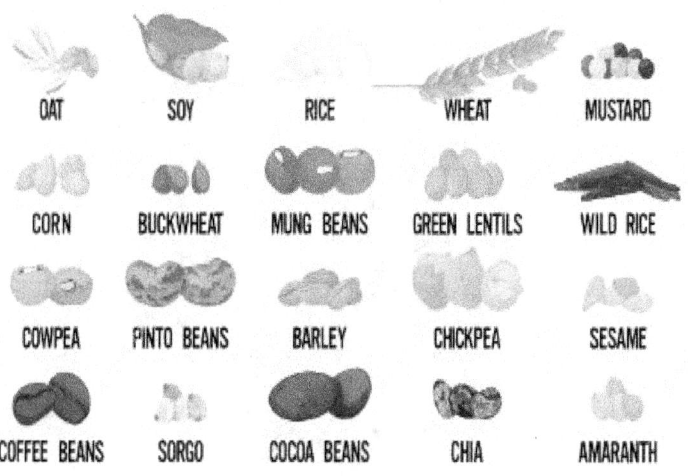

Fiber-rich foods like whole grains can aid in weight management. Fiber helps you feel fuller for longer periods, reducing overall calorie intake and promoting satiety. This can lead to better appetite control and may help prevent overeating, thus supporting weight loss or weight maintenance goals.

Fiber acts as a prebiotic, nourishing beneficial bacteria in the gut and promoting a healthy gut micro biome.

A diverse and balanced gut micro biome is associated with improved digestion, immune function, and overall well-being.

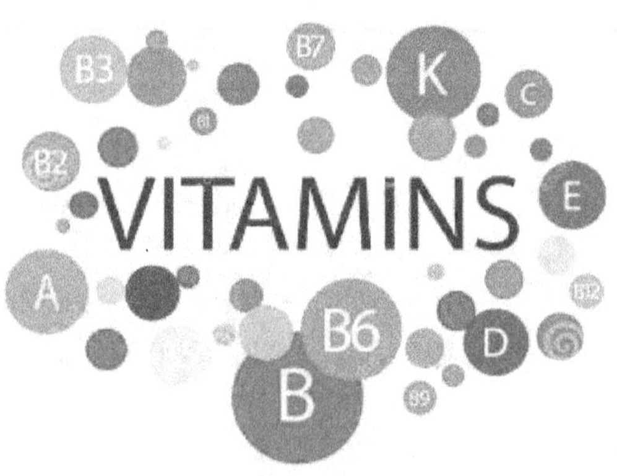

In summary, whole grains and fiber offer numerous health benefits, including improved digestion, heart health, weight management, blood sugar regulation, and gut health. Incorporating whole grain bread and other fiber-rich foods into your diet can contribute to a balanced and nutritious eating pattern that supports overall health and well-being.

Supplements

Vitamin D3: Many people have insufficient levels of vitamin D3, especially those who live in regions with limited sunlight exposure or spend most of their time indoors. Vitamin D3 is essential for bone health, immune function, and mood regulation. Consider taking Vitamin D3 with K2 for absorption, especially during the winter months or if you live in an area or Country or State with limited sun exposure

Vitamin B12: Vitamin B12 is primarily found in animal products, making it essential for vegetarians, vegans, and older adults who may have difficulty absorbing it from food. B12 is crucial for nerve function, DNA synthesis, and red blood cell production. Personally, I opt for a B-12 supplement as I don't consume red meat.

Folic Acid (Folate): Folate is essential for pregnant women or those planning to become pregnant, as it plays a crucial role in fetal development, preventing neural tube defects. Folate is also important for everyone for DNA synthesis and red blood cell formation.

Omega-3 Fatty Acids: I've come to understand the significant role Omega-3 fatty acids play in fat metabolism. Despite the common advice to avoid high-fat foods due to their calorie density and association with weight gain, I've learned that incorporating more Omega-3 rich foods like avocados, nuts and seeds into my diet was actually helping in the fat burning process. By prioritizing these healthy sources of fats, I've found that it has helped me maintain my weight more effectively.

While not a vitamin, omega-3 fatty acids are often supplemented for their numerous health benefits, including heart health, brain function, and reducing inflammation. Fish oil supplements are a common source of omega-3, especially for individuals who don't consume fatty fish regularly.

Calcium: Adequate calcium intake is important for bone health and preventing osteoporosis, especially for postmenopausal women and older adults. However, in order for it to be absorbed into the body, you must be taking it with Magnesium. It's generally recommended to get calcium from dietary sources whenever possible, as excessive calcium supplementation may increase the risk of cardiovascular issues and calcium deposits.

Iron: Iron supplementation may be necessary for people with iron deficiency anemia, particularly women of childbearing age, vegetarians, and those with heavy menstrual cycles. However, excessive iron supplementation can be harmful, so it's essential to have your iron levels checked before starting a supplement regimen.

Multivitamin: A daily multivitamin can help fill nutritional gaps in your diet, especially if you have specific dietary restrictions, limited food choices, or difficulty meeting nutrient needs through food alone. However, a multivitamin should not be used as a substitute for a balanced diet rich in fruits, vegetables, whole grains, and lean proteins.

Before starting any vitamin supplement regimen, it's important to consult with a healthcare provider or registered dietitian to assess your individual needs. Additionally, focus on obtaining essential nutrients from a balanced diet whenever possible, as whole foods provide a wide range of nutrients and beneficial compounds like Fiber, that supplements don't provide.

Chapter 3

Commercial Fad Diets and Surgery

Why start a Diet?

People start diets for a variety of reasons, influenced by both internal and external factors:

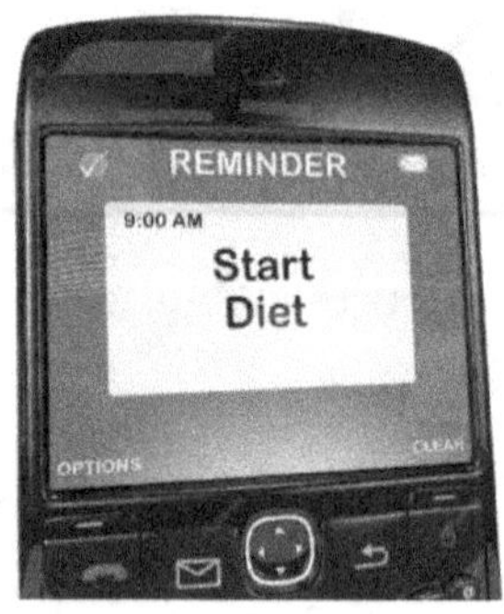

One of the most common reasons people start diets is to manage their weight. Whether they want to lose weight, maintain a healthy weight, or prevent weight gain, dieting is often seen as a way to achieve these goals.

They also have concerns about health issues such as high cholesterol, high blood pressure, diabetes, or other chronic conditions that can prompt individuals to adopt healthier eating habits through dieting. They may aim to improve their overall health or manage specific health conditions through dietary changes.

Societal pressure and personal perceptions of body image can drive people to start diets in pursuit of achieving a certain physique or appearance that aligns with societal standards or personal preferences, such as when you want to pursue in finding your partner that maybe one day you would like to marry, or you want to stand out from the others in a particular career choice.

Some people start diets as part of their fitness journey, aiming to improve athletic performance, build muscle, or enhance physical fitness. They may follow specific dietary plans tailored to their fitness goals, such as increasing protein intake or fueling workouts with specific nutrients. They may have a goal to become a professional bodybuilder.

Peer pressure or social influences, from friends, family members, or coworkers who are dieting or following certain eating trends may motivate some people to start diets. They may feel encouraged or compelled to join others in their dietary pursuits.

Media portrayals of idealized bodies, celebrity diets, and marketing of diet products or programs can influence people to start diets. They may be swayed by promises of quick weight loss, success stories, or endorsements by influencers or celebrities.

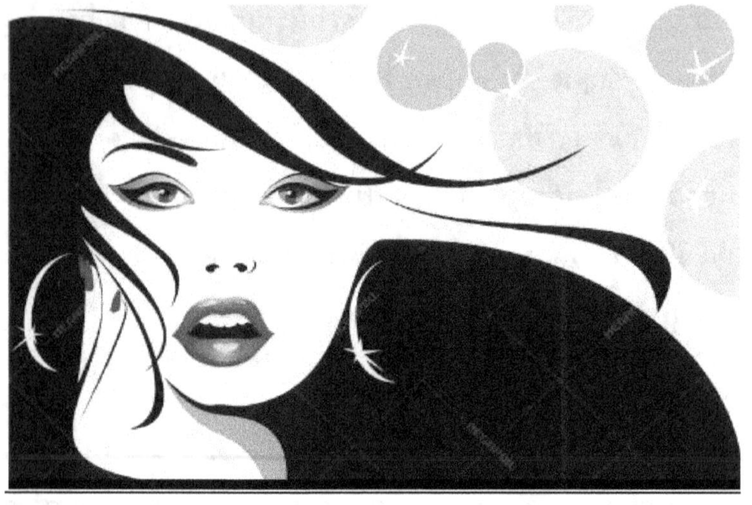

Television commercials showcasing people enthusiastically working out at the gym can also influence people to consider joining a gym.

There are also emotional factors such as stress, boredom, loneliness, or a desire for control may lead people to turn to food restriction or dieting as a coping mechanism. Emotional eating patterns can trigger the initiation of diets as a means of managing emotions or seeking comfort.

Trends in health and wellness, such as popular diets or nutrition trends promoted in the media or on social media platforms, can drive people to try new diets in pursuit of health and well-being.

Overall, the decision to start a diet often has many reasons and is influenced by a combination of personal, social, cultural, and environmental factors. It's important for people to approach dieting with caution, considering their individual needs, preferences, and motivations, and to prioritize overall health and well-being over quick fixes or unrealistic expectations.

Fad Diets

Fad diets are trendy, often extreme eating plans that promise rapid weight loss or other health benefits. They typically gain popularity quickly but are not based on scientific evidence and often lack balance and sustainability. Fad diets often involve restrictive eating patterns, elimination of entire food groups, or reliance on specific foods or supplements.

There are several reasons why fad diets don't work in the long term:

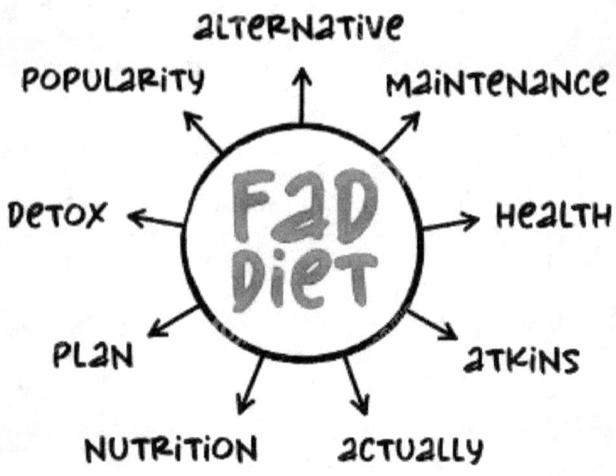

Fad diets often impose extreme and unsustainable restrictions, causing feelings of deprivation and intense cravings. Ultimately, once the diet ends, people tend to regain the weight back. The restrictions often lead to an inability to adhere to the diet and give into cravings.

Many fad diets eliminate entire food groups or severely restrict certain nutrients, leading to nutritional imbalances and deficiencies. This can have negative consequences for overall health and well-being.

Rapid weight loss from fad diets often involves significant calorie restriction, which can slow down metabolism over time. This makes it harder to maintain weight loss and can lead to weight regain once normal eating resumes.

Fad diets are often promoted as one-size-fits-all solutions, failing to consider individual differences in metabolism, lifestyle, preferences, and health needs. What works for one person may not work for another.

Fad diets prioritize short-term results, such as rapid weight loss, over long-term health and sustainability. It often neglects important aspects of overall health, such as physical activity, stress management, and psychological well-being.

Following fad diets can contribute to a cycle of yo-yo dieting, where people, such as I repeatedly lose and regain weight, which can have negative effects on the metabolism, body, and overall health.

Is Surgery a Good choice?

Stomach surgery, also known as bariatric surgery, can be an effective option for weight loss in certain individuals, particularly those who have struggled to lose weight through diet and exercise alone and who have a body mass index (BMI) of 40 or higher, or a BMI of 35 or higher with obesity-related health conditions such as type 2 diabetes or high blood pressure.

There are several types of bariatric surgery. These surgeries work by either reducing the size of the stomach or bypassing a portion of the digestive tract, thereby limiting food intake and/or absorption of calories and nutrients.

Bariatric surgery can lead to significant and sustained weight loss, as well as improvement or resolution of obesity-related health conditions such as type 2 diabetes, high blood pressure, sleep apnea, and joint pain. It can also improve overall quality of life and reduce the risk of premature death associated with obesity.

It is important to note that bariatric surgery is not a quick fix or a one-size-fits-all solution. It requires a lifelong commitment to healthy eating habits, regular exercise, and ongoing medical monitoring. Like any surgical procedure, bariatric surgery carries risks and potential complications, including infection, bleeding, blood clots, nutrient deficiencies, and gastrointestinal issues.

Before considering bariatric surgery, people should undergo a thorough evaluation by a team of healthcare professionals, including a surgeon, dietitian, psychologist, and other_specialists. They should also explore non-surgical weight loss options and fully understand the benefits and potential life threatening risks of surgery.

Ultimately, the decision to undergo bariatric surgery should be made in consultation with a healthcare provider, taking into account individual medical history, lifestyle factors, and treatment goals. It's important to weigh the potential benefits against the risks and to have realistic expectations about the outcomes of surgery.

Chapter 4

Triggers and Anchors

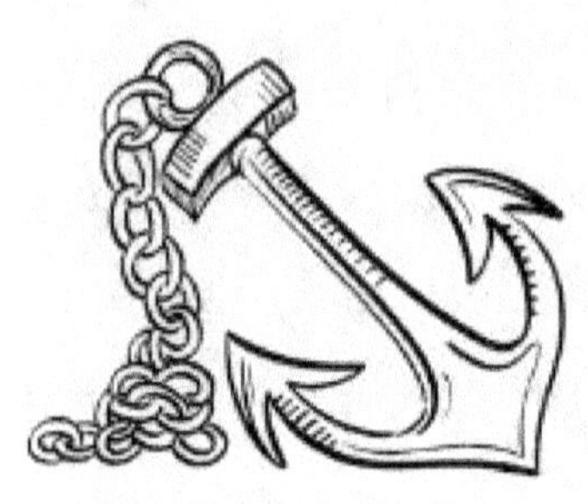

In this book, I aim to teach a concept from psychology that I've learned some time ago, about Triggers, and how it's not always our fault when we give in to temptation and food cravings. A lot of the time it is the subconscious triggers. Our human mind is a complex and intricate system, having both conscious and subconscious processes that influence our thoughts, emotions, and behaviors.

Mental triggers can activate certain thoughts, feelings, or behaviors, usually coming from the subconscious level. These triggers can greatly impact our desires, motivations, and decisions we make, sometimes leading us to want things without fully understanding why.

The subconscious mind plays a significant role in shaping our desires and preferences. While our conscious mind is responsible for rational thought and logical reasoning, the subconscious mind operates beneath the surface, processing information, storing memories, and influencing our perceptions and responses to the world around us.

One of the ways the subconscious mind influences our desires is through the activation of emotional and psychological associations, maybe through images, sounds, smells, or words, which can bring up powerful emotional responses that are deeply ingrained within our subconscious. For example, the sight of a favorite childhood snack might trigger feelings of nostalgia and comfort, leading us to crave it even when we're not hungry, or a song you hear that reminds you of a favorite place or time in your life.

Our subconscious mind can be highly influenced from external factors, including advertising, social norms, and cultural influences. Marketers and advertisers, in particular, are good at finding mental triggers to create desire and promote consumption through cleverly crafted messages, images, and branding strategies. They can tap into our subconscious desires and aspirations, influencing our purchasing decisions without our conscious awareness.

Our subconscious mind is shaped by past experiences, memories, and conditioning, which can influence our desires and behaviors in subtle ways. For example, someone who has experienced trauma or deprivation in childhood may develop subconscious patterns of seeking comfort or security through material possessions or indulgent behaviors, fear of missing out or a desire to belong and fit in.

With all of that being said, I want to share what helped me overcome my sugar cravings.

I used to have a strong fondness for baked goods such as pastries, pies, cakes, and cookies.

When I would walk down a store aisle, I couldn't resist the urge to buy something from the bakery.

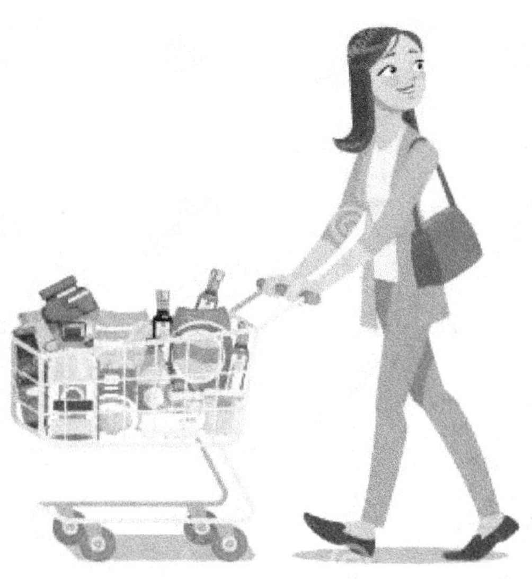

This made it difficult for me to change my eating habits and adopt a healthier diet. After about a week of trying to stay on a new diet that I was trying, I would inevitably give in to temptation and indulge in candy, pastries, or desserts as a reward for myself. However, afterward, I would feel guilty about consuming those treats and would skip lunch or dinner to compensate for the extra calories. This only left me feeling more frustrated because I failed the diet, and I couldn't seem to lose weight.

During this time in my life, I also began reading books and doing research on self improvement strategies in an effort to learn methods to achieve other goals in life. I needed to figure out how to change my thoughts because it became clear negative thoughts were holding me back. This made sense based on what I had learned in psychology years prior. In my research, I was revisiting the concept of triggers and how people are triggered by environmental sources such as commercials, for example. While I already knew about this, I did not know how to change the programming in my mind to reverse the pre-existing psychological triggers.

As I continued to expand my knowledge, I learned how to reverse the triggers that make us do things without thinking. In my case, it was giving in to cravings, and was causing procrastination in different areas of my life.

In my research what I learned was about mental imaging; how to visualize myself physically different, and how to break old habits. This is something that helped me tremendously! I was shocked when I realized I didn't feel tempted to consume or even look at baked goods! They didn't appeal to me anymore and I was able to permanently change my eating habits resulting in weight loss. If I gained any weight back, I knew how to make the changes to take it off right away without feeling deprived.

Here's how it works:

1. Write down why you want to lose weight. Be specific and include details about your reasons. For example, "I want to go to my class reunion and look great," or "I want to feel confident when I look in the mirror."

2. Write down how being overweight makes you feel. Be specific about the emotions it brings up, even if they're uncomfortable.

3. Draw a line down the middle of a piece of paper. On the left side, write "pros," or "positive" and on the right side, write "cons" or "negative."

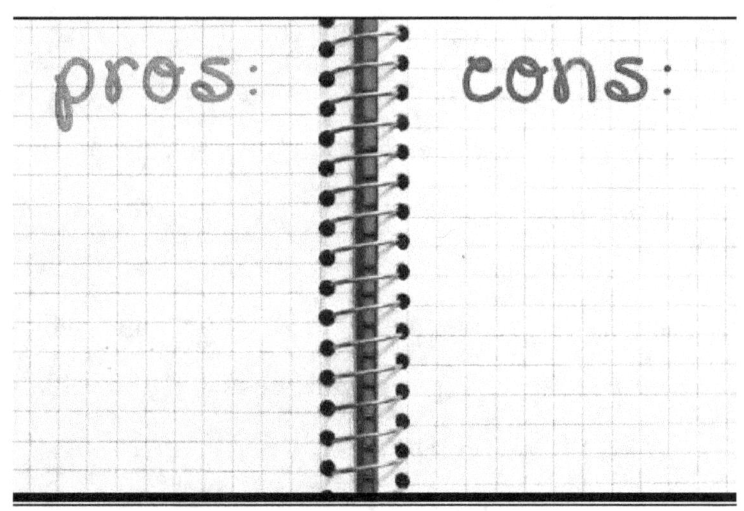

- 4.	List all the reasons why losing weight would be positive (on the left side). On the right side of the page list the negatives of not losing weight and how that would make you feel.

- 5.	Look at your paper. Does one side outweigh the other? If the negative side is longer than the positive side, you clearly have enough reasons to want to make a change.

- 6.	If the list is the same, it means you haven't felt enough pain for your mind and feelings to desire the change.

- In essence, if you can't see or think of enough reasons to change, then your mind won't change. This is how the mind operates. If it's receiving positive rewards even if the rewards are detrimental from not making lifestyle changes, your mind will resist the changes to continue feeling what it considers a positive reward. Your mind will avoid pain and change at all costs if the change is associated with pain.

If you can think of reasons to stay the same, it means you're getting some kind of pleasure or reward from staying in your current state.

After you finish your list and look at your results, if you have more reasons to want the change, you'll move on to the next step. But if your list on the left side is longer or equal to the right side, you still have more reasons to stay where you are.

Your mind hasn't connected enough pain to this change that you're wanting, and this will make it harder to change your mental programming.

Next Step

This process will teach you how to create an anchor.

Do you have a mental Image of how you want to look in your mind? Have you looked into the mirror and said "If I just had a smaller _______." (Fill in the space.) Now imagine how you'd want to look.

Close your eyes and see yourself how you look now and the feeling associated with that thought.   How big does that image look? Is it Big? Now in your mind take that image and shrink it down with your hands as if you are really shrinking it outside your mind. Keep shrinking it down,

down, down, as small as you can. Then take it in your hand, crunch it up, and throw it away into an imaginary trash can.

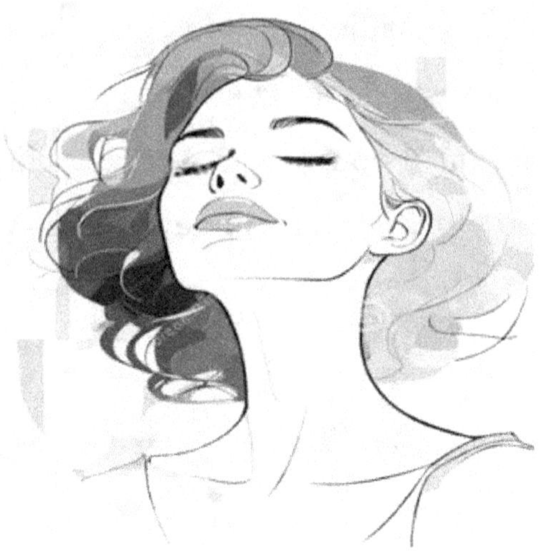

Next, see your own image of how you want to look. If the image is small, make it bigger; make it life size if you can. Feel the feelings of how that makes you feel to see yourself looking the way you want to look and feel. Hold that feeling for a min or so.

Throughout the day, do this visualization in your mind of how you want to look. Envision it as big as possible and feel the emotions associated with that image. Does it make you feel more confident?

Write down how it makes you feel when you see yourself in that way. By jotting down your feelings, you can help reinforce these emotions in your mind. Writing aids in memory retention.

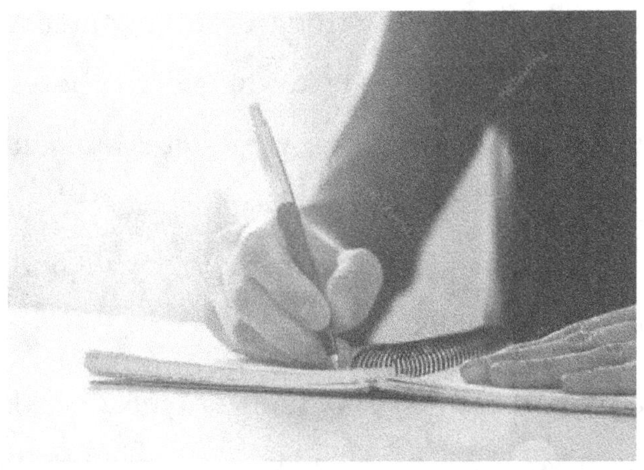

Next, in your mind, visualize whatever is hindering you from reaching your goal weight. Whether it's eating sweets, overeating, eating late at night, or eating due to nervousness or feelings of despair, apply the same visualization technique.

See yourself in your mind doing whatever it is that you want to stop doing. Example: Eating Sweets, eating late at night, binge eating, overeating. Is the picture Big? Make it small. Do the same thing as before. Shrink it down, down, down. As small as you can, then crumble it up and throw it away into the imaginary trash can.

After practicing this a few times a day for a few days, test it out. Try to do the thing that you had a problem with, whatever it was. How do you feel about it now? Do you notice any differences, feeling less attracted to it perhaps? If you still experience a strong desire or intense feelings toward it, then repeat the technique in the same way, maybe for a day or two. Then, try it out again. Once you've made progress with this practice and achieved your desired results, you can always return to it if you find yourself reverting to old habits.

By learning this new method of subconscious mind retraining, you will be able to overcome problem areas related to weight loss. You'll be able to reach your goals without the obstacles that previously hindered your success due to subconscious influences.

Chapter 5

Lifestyles to manage health and weight

Exercise

Exercise is really important for staying healthy and keeping a good weight. When you exercise regularly, it helps your body in many ways. First off, it makes your heart stronger and helps to prevent heart problems like heart disease and strokes. Doing things like walking fast, running, biking, or swimming can make your heart work better, lower your blood pressure, and make your blood flow smoother.

Also, exercise helps to keep you from gaining too much weight .When you eat healthy and exercise a lot, your body burns up extra calories and makes it easier to keep a good weight. Plus, exercising builds up your muscles, which not only makes you look more toned but also helps your body burn calories even when you're not doing anything. In other words, having more muscle helps keep fat off.

Besides making your body stronger, exercise is good for your brain too. When you work out, your brain releases chemicals called endorphins, which make you feel happy and calm. This helps reduce stress, anxiety, and sadness, and makes you feel better overall. Regular exercise has also been shown to help with sleep, thinking better, and feeling good about yourself.

Exercise also keeps your bones strong and helps prevent them from getting weak as you get older. Things like walking, running, and lifting weights help your bones stay strong and less likely to break, especially when you're older.

In short, doing exercise every day is super important for staying healthy and keeping a good weight. You can do all kinds of things to stay active, like going to the gym, playing outside, or even just taking the stairs instead of the elevator. Finding ways to move more can really help your heart, your weight, and your mood, making you feel better and healthier overall.

Muscle and strength training

Having muscles and doing strength training exercises are really good for losing weight, keeping it off, and keeping your bones strong. When you have muscles, they help you burn calories, even when you're not doing anything. So, having more muscle makes it easier to burn calories and stay at a healthy weight.

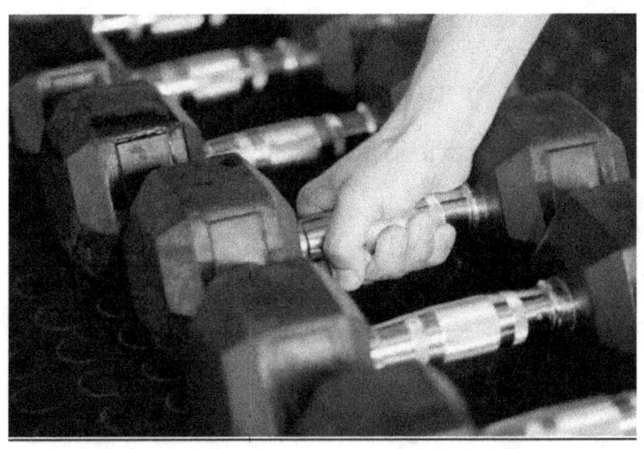

Strength training exercises are things like lifting weights, using resistance bands, or doing exercises with just your body weight. These exercises help you build and keep your muscle mass. When you do strength training regularly, you can make your muscles stronger and help your body burn calories better. This makes it easier to stay at a healthy weight over time.

Also, strength training is important for keeping your bones strong and preventing a condition called osteoporosis. Osteoporosis happens when your bones become weak and can break easily. As people get older, their bones naturally become less dense, which makes them more likely to get osteoporosis. But when you do exercises that put stress on your bones, like strength training, it helps make them stronger and less likely to break. This is really important for staying healthy as you get older.

Doing strength training exercises also makes it easier to do everyday activities and lowers your risk of getting hurt. When your muscles are strong, you can move around better and have less chance of falling or getting hurt. This is especially important as you get older and might have more trouble moving around.

What exercise type is best?

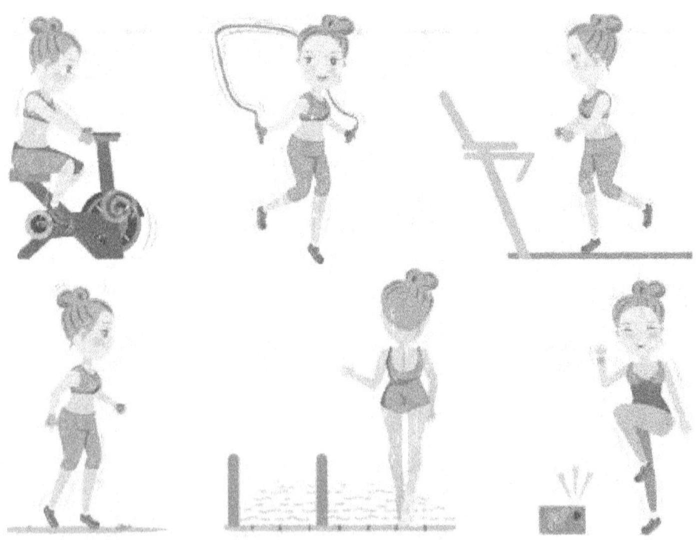

Deciding which exercise to do—cardio, strength training, or both—depends on what you want to achieve with your fitness and what you like doing. Each type of exercise has its own benefits and helps you stay healthy and fit.

Cardio exercises, also known as cardiovascular exercises, are good for your heart health, endurance, and burning calories. They include things like running, biking, swimming, and brisk walking. When you do cardio, your heart rate goes up, pumping more blood and oxygen to your muscles and organs. Doing cardio regularly can lower your risk of heart disease, reduce blood pressure, and improve your cholesterol levels. It's also great for losing weight and making you feel happier because it releases endorphins, which are natural chemicals that make you feel good.

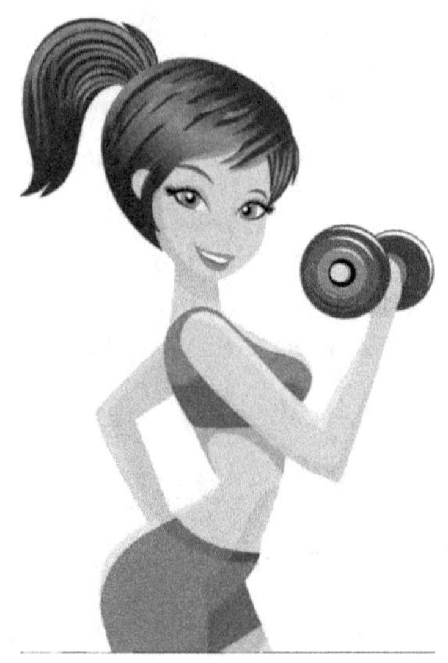

Strength training, on the other hand, focuses on making your muscles stronger and more toned by using weights, resistance bands, or doing exercises like push-ups and squats. Strength training helps you build muscle, make your bones stronger, and boost your metabolism. It also improves your overall strength, balance, and how well you can move, which lowers your chances of getting hurt. Plus, it can make you feel better about your body by making your muscles look more defined and your appearance more toned.

Even though cardio and strength training are different, doing both together can give you the best results for your health and fitness. Doing strength training as a cardio workout lets you enjoy the benefits of having a healthy heart, strong muscles, and better weight management. And doing different exercises keeps things interesting and fun, so you're more likely to stick with it.

Something different to try is a weight training cardio workout. It can be a great way to get your heart pumping and improve your cardiovascular health. This is where you do Sets with weights, but instead of resting 5 min you rest about 20 seconds and you continue to the next exercise.

 While it might not seem like traditional cardio exercises such as running or cycling, weight training still gets your heart rate up and makes you breathe harder. When you lift weights, your muscles need more oxygen, and your heart has to work harder to deliver it. This increases your heart rate, similar to how it does during cardio exercises.

One of the benefits of weight training as a cardio workout is that it not only strengthens your muscles but also provides a cardiovascular challenge. Doing exercises like squats, lunges, or lifting weights quickly in a circuit can elevate your heart rate and improve your endurance. This type of workout not only burns calories during the session but also keeps your metabolism elevated afterward, helping with weight loss and management.

Additionally, weight training offers the advantage of building lean muscle mass, which can further enhance your metabolism and calorie-burning potential. As you build more muscle, your body becomes more efficient at burning calories, even at rest. This can contribute to long-term weight management and overall health improvement.

Incorporating weight training into your fitness routine alongside traditional cardio exercises can provide a well-rounded approach to fitness. By challenging your cardiovascular system while also building strength and muscle mass, you can improve your overall health, fitness, and body composition. Plus, weight training adds variety to your workouts, making them more enjoyable and sustainable in the long run.

Whether you're lifting weights at the gym, using resistance bands at home, or doing bodyweight exercises, incorporating weight training as part of your cardio routine can offer numerous benefits for your health and well-being.

Chapter 6

Healthy Diet Basics

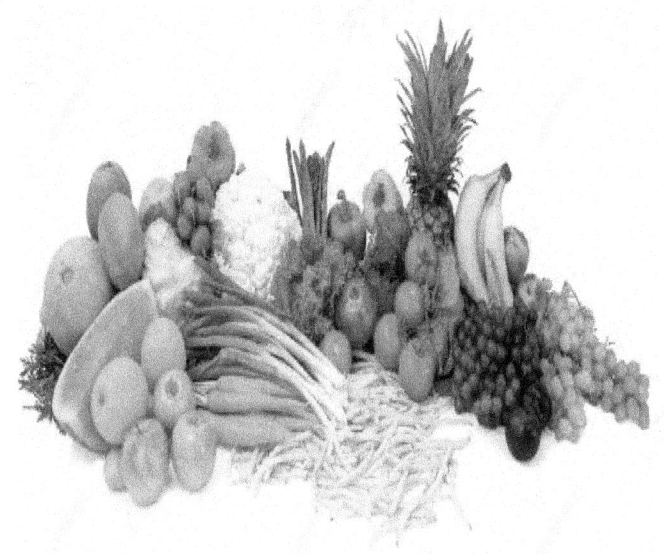

What to eat?

Eating a variety of basic foods is important for maintaining good health and providing your body with the nutrients it needs to function properly. Here are some basic foods that we should include in our diet and why they are beneficial:

Fruits and vegetables: Fruits and vegetables are rich in vitamins, minerals, and antioxidants that support overall health and reduce the risk of chronic diseases such as heart disease, stroke, and certain cancers. They are also high in fiber, which aids in digestion and helps to_keep you feeling full, making it easier to maintain a healthy weight.

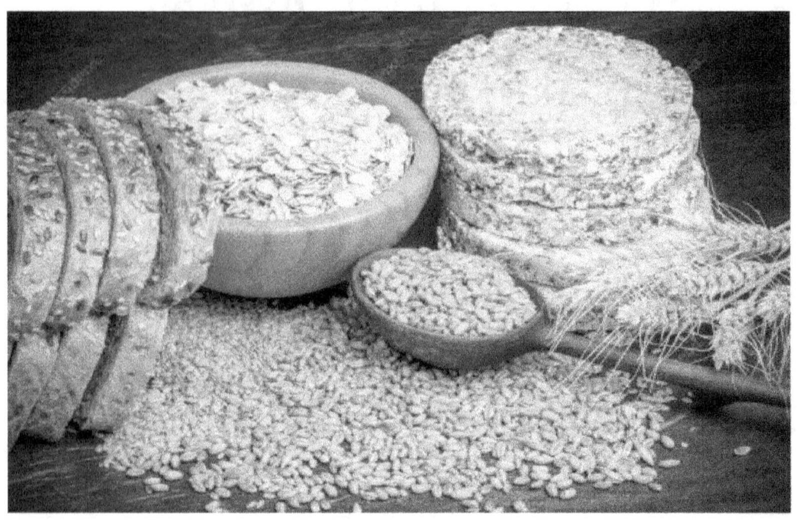

Whole grains: Whole grains like oats, brown rice, quinoa, and whole wheat provide essential nutrients like fiber, vitamins, and minerals. They also help to regulate blood sugar levels, reduce the risk of heart disease, and support digestive health.

Lean proteins: Lean protein sources such as chicken, turkey, fish, beans, lentils, and tofu are important for building and repairing tissues, muscles, and organs. They also help to keep you feeling full and satisfied, making it easier to control your appetite and maintain a healthy weight.

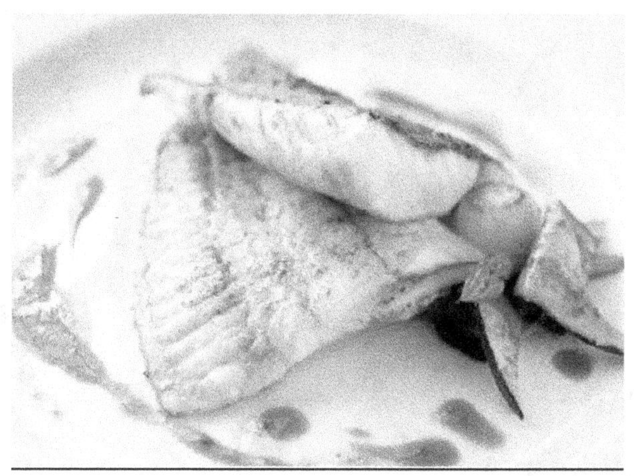

Dairy or dairy alternatives: Dairy products like milk, yogurt, and cheese are rich in calcium, which is essential for building and maintaining strong bones and teeth. If you're lactose intolerant or if you have allergies or maybe just prefer plant-based options, you can choose dairy alternatives like almond milk, soy milk, or fortified plant-based yogurts.

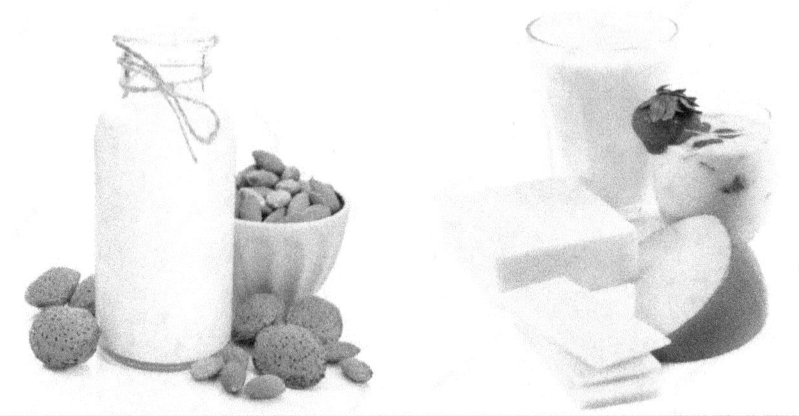

Healthy fats

What I've come to learn over the last few years, which is really exciting, is that healthy fats found in foods like nuts, seeds, avocados, and olive oil, actually help to burn fat and help the body lose weight. Yes, it's the omega fatty acids that help do this. Adding nuts, seeds, or avocado to a salad or in your meals gives you that extra edge to burn more fat. These amino acids are also essential for brain health, hormone production, and absorbing fat-soluble vitamins. They also help to reduce inflammation and lower the risk of heart disease when consumed in moderation.

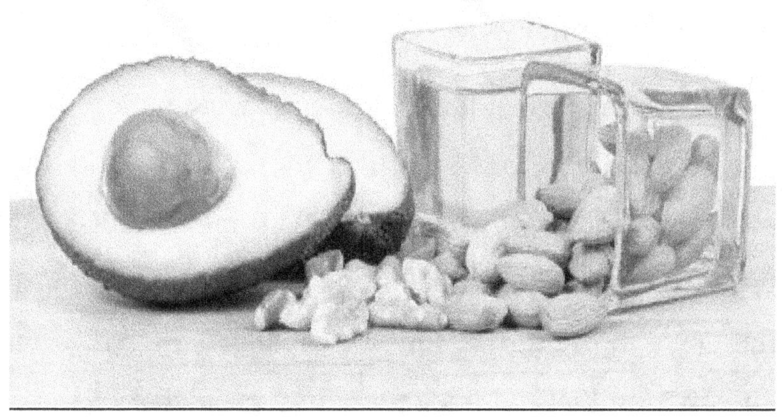

By including these basic foods in your diet regularly, you can ensure that your body receives the essential nutrients it needs to thrive. Aim to eat a variety of foods from each food group to ensure you get a wide range of nutrients and enjoy better overall health and well-being.

What amount of Food to eat.

Figuring out your calorie level

Over the years, I've found it challenging to follow diet plans from the various books I've used, because they often recommend foods that I can't eat. One issue is my intolerance to dairy, which is commonly included in many diets. However, nowadays, there are non-dairy alternatives available. Another problem I face is that I don't consume much meat; I prefer eating only chicken and fish. A lot of the meals would revolve the meal plans around meats I didn't eat, or include dairy which I couldn't have.

Because of this, I couldn't stick to a preset diet plan; I chose to count calories instead. I thought it would allow me to eat what I liked while staying within my daily calorie limit. However, this approach wasn't successful, because I often ate calorie-dense foods, reaching my daily limit before dinner. I lacked understanding of which foods to eat and how to regulate my eating habits.

Years later, with much failure in managing my weight, I figured out what types of food to eat and how much to eat by following a plan based on calories and portion sizes. It worked well for me because, considering my height and weight, I'm supposed to consume fewer calories than someone who is twice my weight and height.

To figure out your calorie level based on your weight, you can use a basic formula to estimate your Total Daily Energy Expenditure (TDEE), which represents the total number of calories your body burns in a day.

Adjust based on weight goals: If you're looking to lose weight, you'll want to create a calorie deficit by consuming fewer calories than your TDEE. A deficit of 500-1000 calories per day can lead to a safe and sustainable weight loss of about 1-2 pounds per week. Conversely, if you're looking to gain weight, you'll want to consume more calories than your TDEE to create a surplus.

A Multiply your current weight in pounds x 11

B. Take your calorie baseline + 400 this will give you your caloric needs

C. Minus your caloric needs by 750 (Caloric Deficit) this will give you your calorie target.

If your number is less than 1,200 round up to 1,200 if it's more that 2,300 round down to 2,000

Here is an Example of how much to eat for 1,200 calories a day.

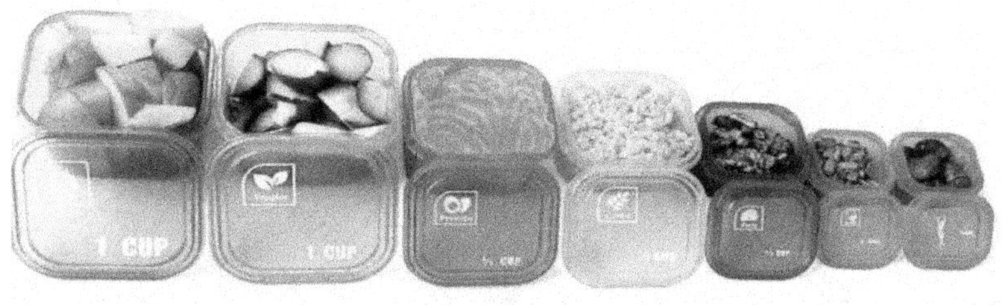

Get Containers at Amazon with this Link

https://amzn.to/3WlgPYA

3 – 1 cup purple container servings of Fruit

2 – 1 cup green container servings of vegetables

4 - ¾ cup red container servings of Meat

2 -½ cup yellow container servings of Starch Carbohydrates

1 - ¼ cup blue container healthy Fats

2 - Tbsp orange container seeds or nuts

2 - Tbsp orange container cooking oil

For a 1,500-1,700 Calorie plan

 4- C of veggies, 3- C of fruit   4- ¾ C Meat   3- C Starchy Carb

And 4 Tbs Oil Everything else stays the same as 1200 cal plan

For a 1,800 – 2,099 Calorie plan

5-C of veggies, 5 - ¾ C meat, 4- C Starchy Carbs

3 Tbsp of Oil Everything else stays the same as 1200 Calorie plan

 For a 2,100 – 2,300 Calorie Plan

6- C of veggies, 4- C fruit, 6- ¾ C meat, 4- C Starchy Carbs

6 Tbsp of Oil Everything else stays the same as 1,200 Calorie plan

Using Portion control is a great way to estimate how much food your eating in a day.   This really helped me to know how much food I should

Be eating, so that I didn't over excess starchy carbs when trying to reduce my weight.

A list of some healthy starches

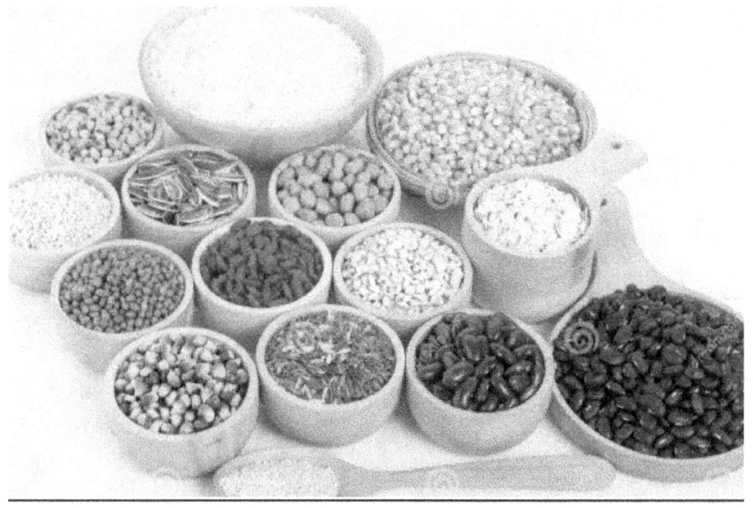

1.   Potatoes (including white, sweet, and red potatoes)

2.   Corn (including cornmeal and popcorn)

3. Rice (including white, brown, and wild rice)

4. Pasta (including spaghetti, macaroni, and penne)

5. Bread (including whole wheat, white, and rye bread)

6. Cereal (including oatmeal, corn flakes, and bran flakes)

7. Quinoa

8. Barley

9. Bulgur

10. Millet

11. Amaranth

12. Buckwheat

13. Plantains

14. Winter squash (including butternut squash and acorn squash)

15. Legumes (including beans, lentils, and chickpeas)

A list of some unhealthy starches

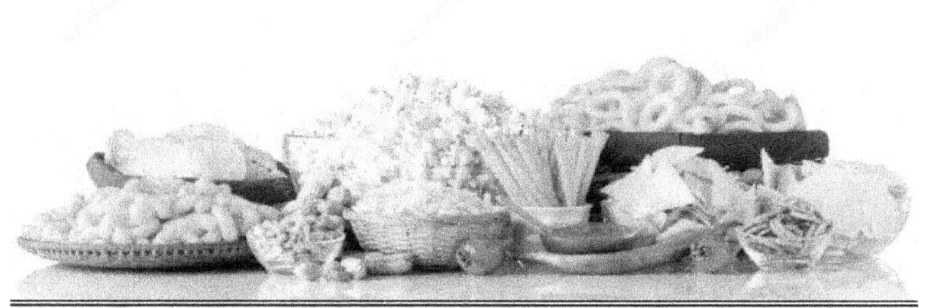

1. White bread

2. White rice

3. Regular pasta

4. Pastries (such as croissants, doughnuts, and Danishes)

5. Sugary breakfast cereals

6. White potatoes (especially when fried or processed)

7. Instant mashed potatoes

8. Processed snack foods (such as potato chips and pretzels)

9. Sugary snacks (such as cakes, cookies, and muffins)

10. Sweetened beverages (such as soda, fruit juices, and energy drinks)

11. Highly processed grains (such as white flour and white rice)

12. Sugary desserts (such as ice cream, candy bars, and chocolate)

On a calorie diet, it's important to pay attention to portion sizes to ensure you're getting the right balance of nutrients while still meeting your calorie goals. Here's a basic alternative guide to portion sizes for meat, vegetables, and carbohydrates/starches:

Here's an alternative approach you can consider, focusing on portion management

Meat/protein: Aim to include a palm-sized portion of lean protein with each meal, such as chicken breast, turkey, fish, tofu, or lean cuts of beef or pork. A palm-sized portion is roughly equivalent to 3-4 ounces, or about the size and thickness of your palm. This provides your body with essential amino acids for muscle repair and growth while keeping your calorie intake in check.

Vegetables: Fill half of your plate with non-starchy vegetables like leafy greens, broccoli, bell peppers, carrots, and cucumbers. These vegetables are low in calories and high in fiber, vitamins, and minerals, making them ideal for weight loss and overall health. Aim to include at least 2-3 servings of vegetables with each meal, which can be equivalent to 1-2 cups of raw vegetables or 1/2 to 1 cup of cooked vegetables.

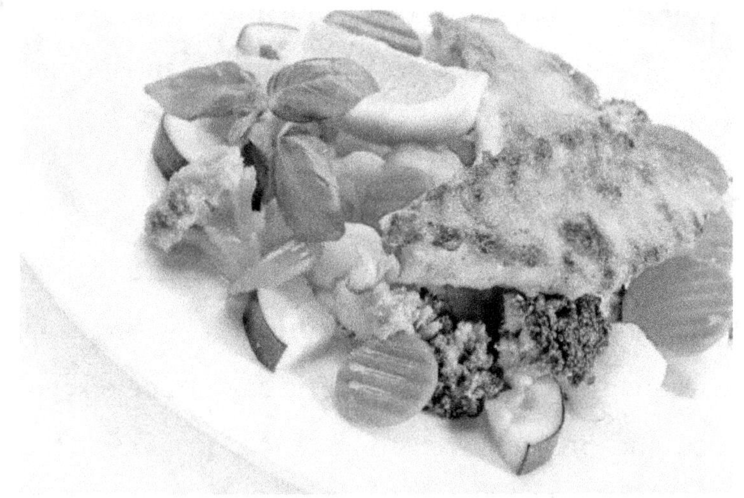

Carbohydrates/starches: Opt for whole grains and complex carbohydrates to provide sustained energy and fiber. Include 1-2 servings of carbohydrates/starches with each meal, such as whole grain bread, brown rice, quinoa, sweet potatoes, or legumes. A serving size is typically equivalent to 1/2 to 1 cup cooked or 1 slice of bread. Be mindful of portion sizes to avoid overeating and exceeding your calorie goals.

Keep in mind that these calculations provide estimates, and individual factors such as metabolism, muscle mass, and genetics can influence calorie needs. It's also essential to listen to your body's hunger and fullness cues and adjust your calorie intake based on your activity level, goals, and overall health. If you're unsure about how to determine your calorie needs or create nutrition plan, consider consulting with a registered dietitian or nutritionist for personalized guidance.

When to Eat

Remember to listen to your body's hunger and fullness cues and adjust portion sizes accordingly. Eating smaller, more frequent meals throughout the day can help keep you satisfied and prevent overeating. And don't forget to stay hydrated by drinking plenty of water throughout the day to support digestion and overall well-being.

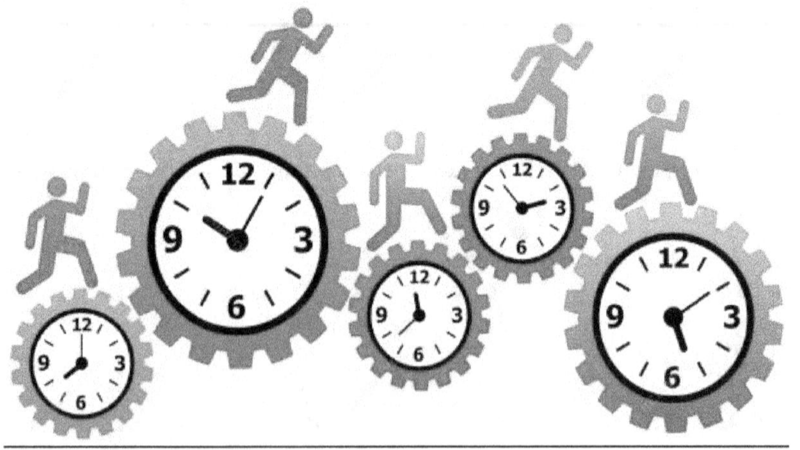

The timing of meals during the day can affect your health and how you feel. Although there isn't one right time for everyone to eat, there are some general ideas to think about.

Breakfast: Many people suggest eating a good breakfast to wake up your body and give you energy for the day. It's best to eat breakfast a few hours after waking up to fill up your energy stores after not eating all night. A healthy breakfast could have things like protein, good fats, and carbs to keep you full and focused until your next meal.

Mid-Morning Snack: You may feel hungry or need a boost in the morning. If that's you, having a small snack around mid-morning could be helpful. Snacks like fruit, nuts, or low fat cottage cheese can give you some nutrients and keep hunger away until lunch.

Lunch: Eating lunch around midday or early afternoon helps give your body more energy for the rest of the day. A balanced lunch with protein, veggies, whole grains, and good fats can keep you full until dinner.

Afternoon Snack: Like the mid-morning snack, having a small snack in the afternoon can be good for keeping hunger away. Veggies with hummus, yogurt with fruit, or a handful of trail mix can be good choices to hold you over until dinner.

Dinner: Having dinner a few hours before bedtime gives your body time to digest before sleep. A balanced dinner with protein, veggies, and carbs gives your body the nutrients it needs and can help you sleep better. It's best to avoid heavy, rich foods close to bedtime, as they might make it harder to sleep well.

Overall, when you eat depends on you and how you feel. Paying attention to when you're hungry and full and eating regular meals and snacks can help keep your energy levels steady and support your health.

Conclusion

In conclusion, my successful weight management journey was achieved through a combination of strategies including building muscle, exercising three to five days a week, cutting sugars, and practicing portion control.

I also practiced eliminating triggers by doing mental imaging work to help with sugar cravings. Reducing sugar intake, particularly from processed foods and sugary beverages, helped me to control calorie consumption, stabilize sugar levels, and promote weight loss.

Building muscle through strength training exercises helped to increase my metabolism and improve my body composition. Exercising three to five days a week, incorporating a cardiovascular strength training workout, played a vital role in burning calories, getting a stronger body, and enhancing my overall well-being.

Additionally, practicing portion control by being mindful of serving sizes and listening to hunger and fullness cues allowed me to manage calorie intake effectively and prevent overeating.

Overall, by incorporating these strategies into my lifestyle consistently, I not only achieved my weight loss goals but also successfully maintained my weight over time. This underscores the importance of adopting a holistic approach to weight management, focusing on building muscle, exercising regularly, cutting sugars, and practicing portion control for long-term success in achieving and maintaining a healthy weight.

If you found this book helpful, I'd be very appreciative if you left a favorable review on Amazon!

www.ingramcontent.com/pod-product-compliance
Lightning Source LLC
Chambersburg PA
CBHW051652250726
48653CB00007B/2626